**Take Care
of Yourself**

Staying
Healthy

by Ashley Richardson

PEBBLE
a capstone imprint

Published by Pebble, an imprint of Capstone.
1710 Roe Crest Drive, North Mankato, Minnesota 56003
capstonepub.com

Library of Congress Cataloging-in-Publication Data
Names: Richardson, Ashley, author.
Title: Staying healthy / by Ashley Richardson.
Description: North Mankato, Minnesota : Pebble, [2022] | Series: Take care of yourself | Includes bibliographical references and index. | Audience: Ages 5–8 | Audience: Grades K–1 | Summary: "Everyone gets sick sometimes, but there are lots of ways to take good care of oneself. Readers learn the importance of hand washing, sleep, mental health, diet, and exercise. People who can help readers stay healthy are also described" —Provided by publisher.
Identifiers: LCCN 2021029990 (print) | LCCN 2021029991 (ebook) | ISBN 9781663976802 (hardcover) | ISBN 9781666325553 (paperback) | ISBN 9781666325560 (pdf) | ISBN 9781666325584 (kindle edition)
Subjects: LCSH: Health—Juvenile literature. | Hygiene—Juvenile literature.
Classification: LCC RA777 .R54 2022 (print) | LCC RA777 (ebook) | DDC 613—dc23
LC record available at https://lccn.loc.gov/2021029990
LC ebook record available at https://lccn.loc.gov/2021029991

Image Credits
Getty Images: Brothers91, 12, Maskot, 9; Shutterstock: Anna Golant (design element) throughout, Edward_Maslennikov, 21 (paper, markers), Gorynvd, 11, Jet Cat Studio, 17, jittawit21, 7, Krakenimages.com, 15, LightField Studios, 5, LightField Studios, 6, Monkey Business Images, 18, paulaphoto, 19, PEPPERSMINT, Cover, Pixel-Shot, 8, Rido, 13, Seregam, 21 (ruler)

Editorial Credits
Editor: Erika L. Shores; Designer: Heidi Thompson; Media Researcher: Jo Miller; Production Specialist: Tori Abraham

All internet sites appearing in back matter were available and accurate when this book was sent to press.

Printed and bound in the USA. PO4608

Table of Contents

Words in **bold** are in the glossary.

Love Your Body

Your body does amazing things every day. Arms help you swing a baseball bat. Eyes help you watch movies. Your brain helps you imagine. There are many reasons to love your body and keep it healthy.

Get enough sleep. Exercise. Eat healthy foods. Healthy bodies can fight off **germs** and illness. Healthy bodies are strong.

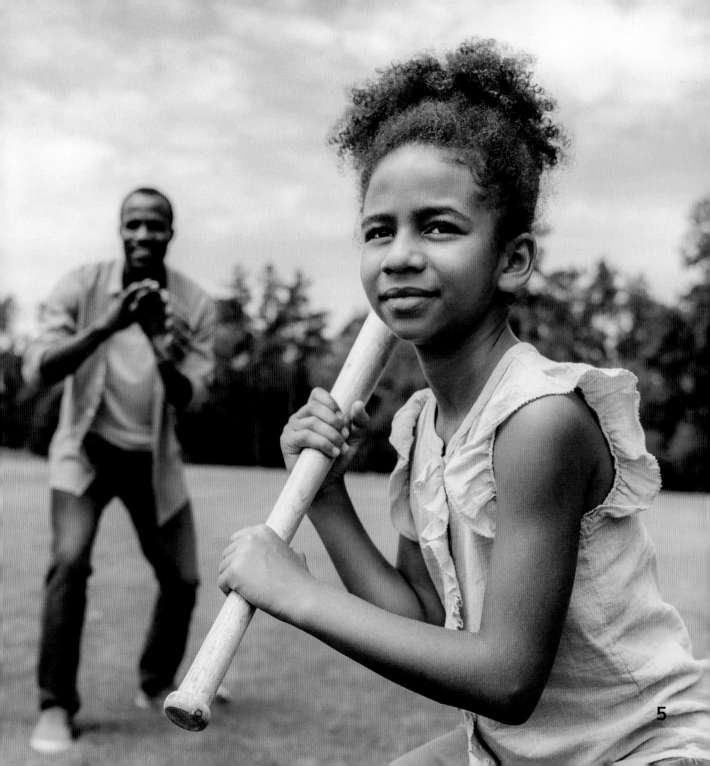

Getting Enough Sleep

Sleep is important to a healthy body. Sleep will help you feel good during the day. Sleep helps you stay focused in school. You may feel more **social**. Sleep even helps your body heal.

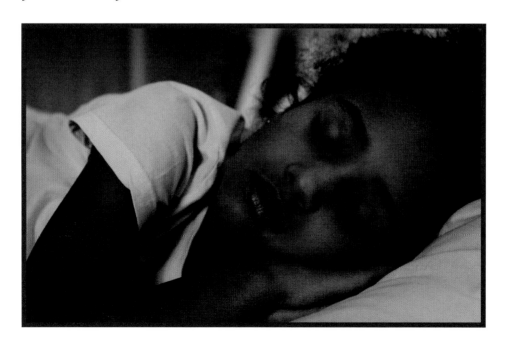

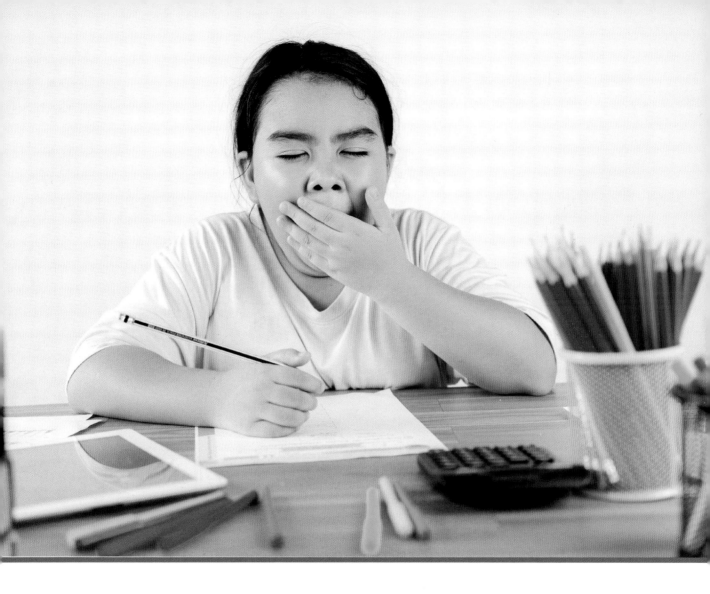

Sometimes people feel grumpy without enough sleep. Kids need 9 to 12 hours of sleep every night. Are you getting enough?

Staying Active

Run. Jump. Leap! Be active for at least one hour every day. Physical activity keeps your body healthy. Physical activity even makes "happy" chemicals in the brain. These chemicals are called **endorphins**.

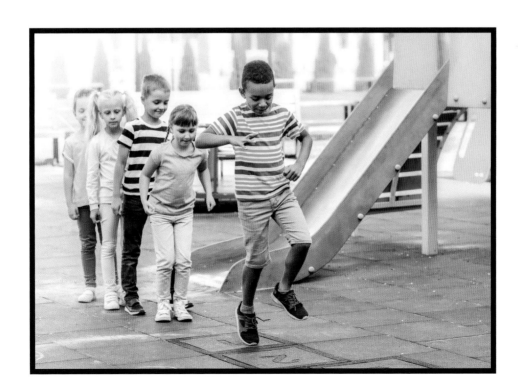

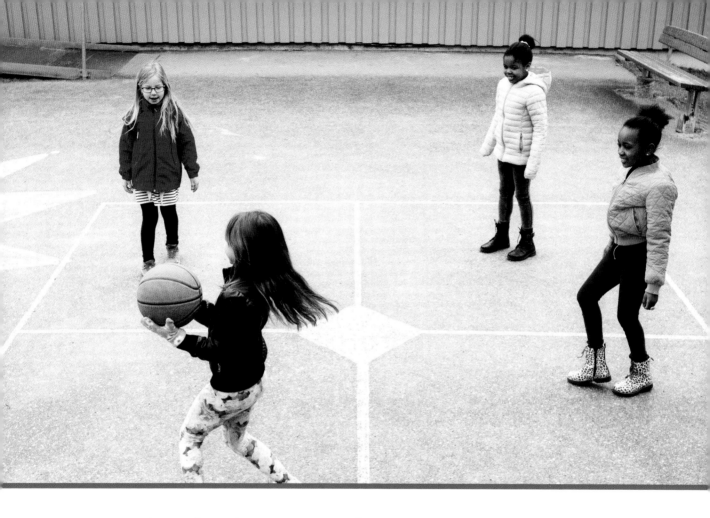

At school, you can play games with friends during recess. Physical education teachers can also show you fun activities. Maybe you can teach your family the same activity at home.

Fuel Your Body

Food is fuel for the body. Food gives you energy. Eat brown rice and other grains. Fish and meat help build muscles. Vegetables and fruits are full of **nutrients**. Water helps your body work properly. Drink five glasses of water every day.

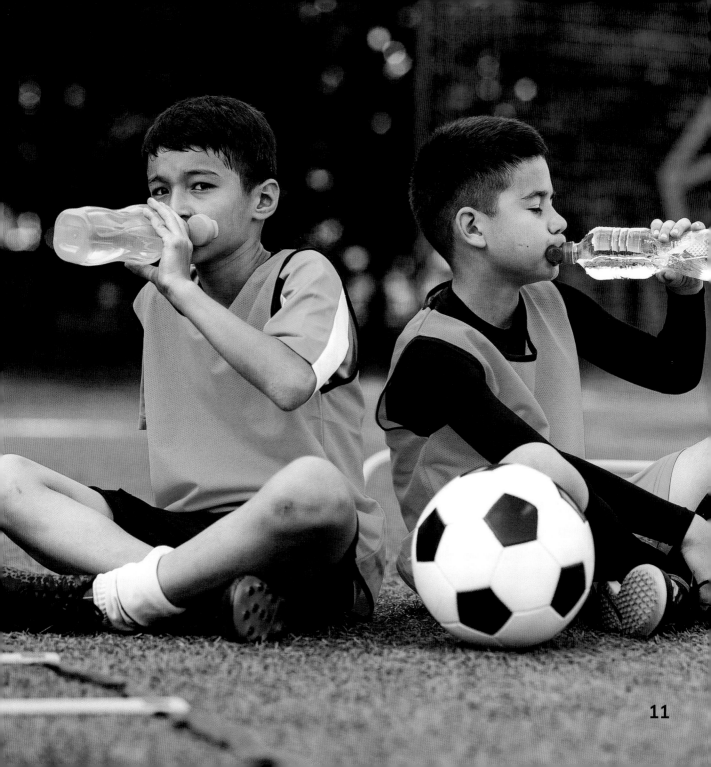

Fighting Off Germs

Germs are too small to see. They enter the body through the eyes, nose, and mouth. To fight off germs, avoid touching your face. Wash your hands with soap and warm water for at least 20 seconds.

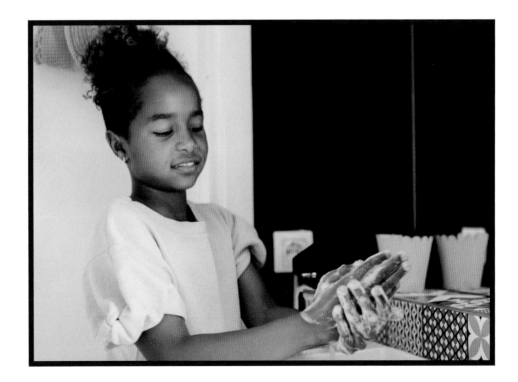

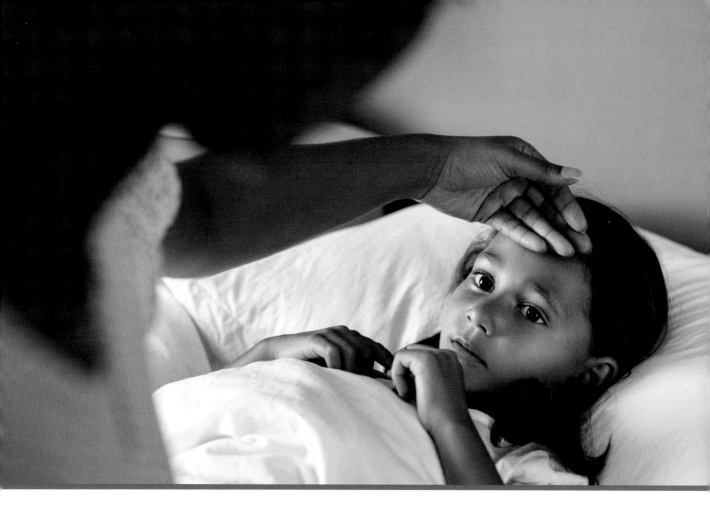

Help others stay healthy. Sneeze or cough into a tissue or your elbow. Stay home when you're sick. Or see a doctor if you need medicine. These **habits** help stop the spread of germs.

A Healthy Mind

You care for your body. Care for your mind too. Drinking lots of water and eating healthy are important for brain power. What else can you feed your mind? Feed your mind positive thoughts and kind words. Think kindly about yourself. What are you proud of today?

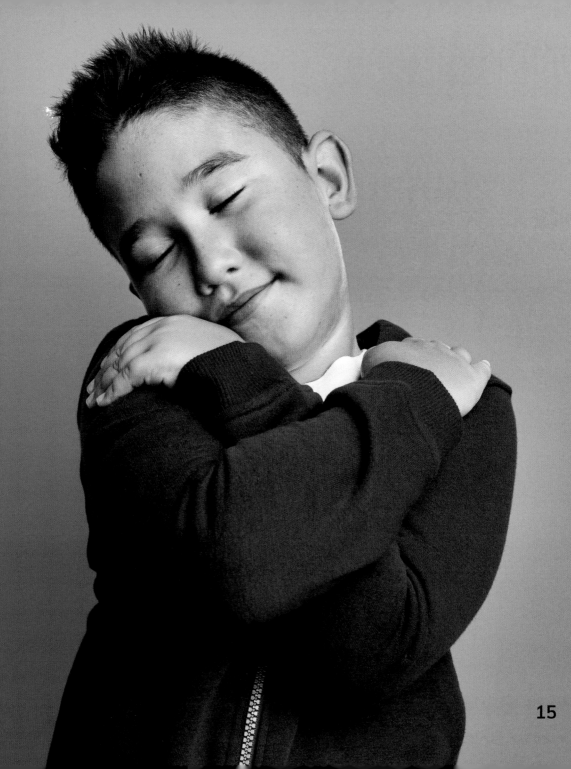

Self-Care

Staying healthy is a way to show your mind and body love. It means you are practicing self-care. Self-care means paying attention to what your body needs. Drink water when you're thirsty. Go to bed early when you're tired. See a doctor when you're sick. These are all kinds of self-care.

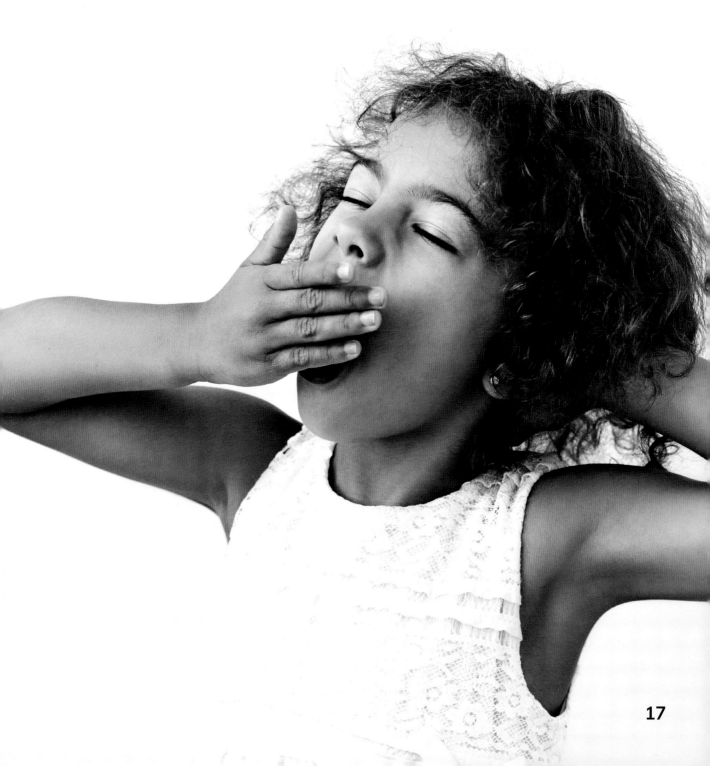

Sometimes we need other people to help us with our care. Everyone has sad or worried feelings at times. But sometimes they don't go away. A **therapist** can help you with your feelings. If you need help eating healthy, you and a family member can talk to a **nutritionist**.

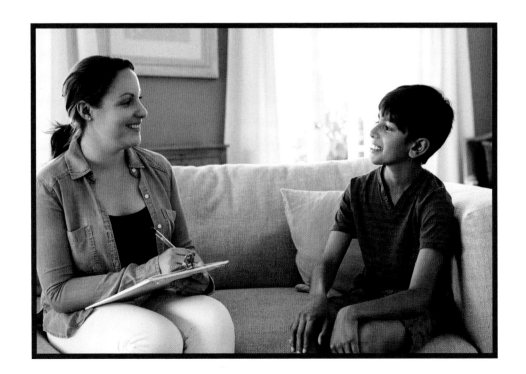

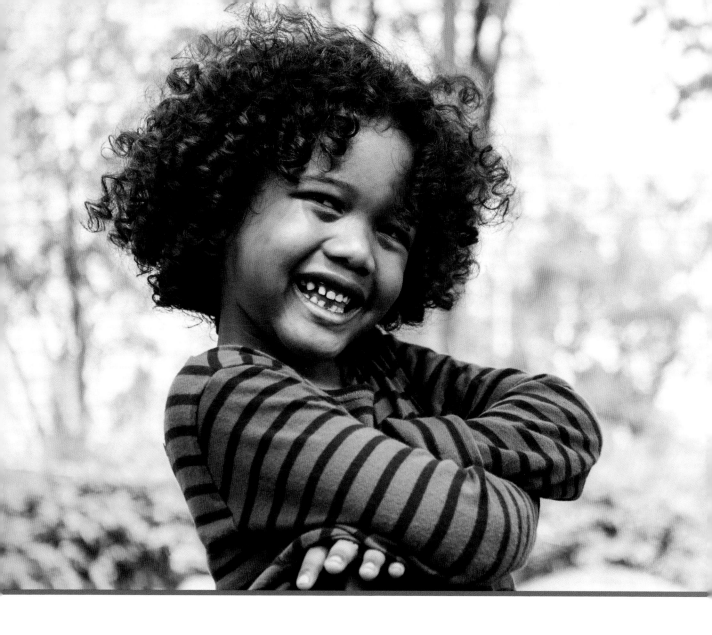

You can take care of yourself. Celebrate
your healthy and happy body!

Plan a Healthy Day

There are many things that help keep us healthy. Exercise, sleep, healthy food, and even good deeds. Let's create a plan for a healthy day.

What You Need:

- blank piece of paper
- pencil, markers, or crayons
- ruler

What You Do:

1. On the piece of paper, draw a big circle.
2. Split the circle into four even parts. In one part, write "Exercise." In another part, write "Healthy Food." In the next part, write "Sleep." In the last part, write "Kindness."

3. Now, pick one goal for each section. Maybe for "Exercise" you want to play soccer for one hour. Maybe in "Kindness" you want to make a card for a friend. Pick a goal for each section. Draw a picture to go with it.

4. Follow your plan for the day.

Glossary

endorphin (en-DOR-fin)—a natural chemical in the body that helps fight pain; they also can make people feel happy

germ (JURM)—a tiny living thing that can cause disease

habit (HAB-it)—something that you do often

nutrient (NOO-tree-uhnt)—substances, such as vitamins, that plants, animals, and people need for good health

nutritionist (noo-TRISH-uhn-ist)—a person who studies and is an expert on food and healthy eating

social (SOH-shuhl)—enjoying other people

therapist (THER-uh-pist)—a person who is trained in helping people talk through and deal with their emotions

Read More

Lindeen, Mary. *Being Kind to Yourself*. Chicago: Norwood House Press, 2021.

MacReady, R. J. *Eating Healthy Foods*. New York: Cavendish Square Publishing, 2022.

Rustad, Martha E. H. *Care for Your Body*. North Mankato, MN: Capstone, 2020.

Internet Sites

Food Hero
foodhero.org/kids

Health for Kids: Sneezing, Coughs, and Colds
healthforkids.co.uk/staying-healthy/sneezing-coughs-and-colds/

Index

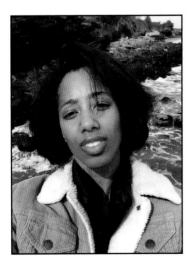

About the Author

Ashley Richardson writes fiction, poetry, and creative nonfiction. She enjoys reading all kinds of books and lives in the Midwest with a houseful of plants. For fun, Ashley loves to inline skate in the park.